Distribution, publication, and copying in any form are prohibited and subject to damages.

TEN HYPNOSES

Copying, publishing, and sharing with third parties are only permitted with the written consent of the author. Please observe the notes on copyright and usage.

Distribution, publication, and copying in any form are prohibited and subject to damages.

Copying, publishing, and sharing with third parties are only permitted with the written consent of the author. Please observe the notes on copyright and usage.

Distribution, publication, and copying in any form are prohibited and subject to damages.

Ingo Michael Simon

TEN HYPNOSES

16

Post-Traumatic Stress

Copying, publishing, and sharing with third parties are only permitted with the written consent of the author. Please observe the notes on copyright and usage.

Distribution, publication, and copying in any form are prohibited and subject to damages.

© 2024 Ingo Michael Simon
All rights reserved.
Independently published
www.ingosimon.com

Important Notes for Urgent Attention:
The contents of this book are based on the practical experiences of the author with hypnosis applications and psychotherapy in a trance state. Although the author has strived for the utmost care, errors or misunderstandings in the presentation cannot be completely excluded. Therapeutic work with people and the application of hypnosis are solely the responsibility of the hypnotist. It cannot be ruled out that parts of this book may be misunderstood or that the application of a presented procedure may cause an undesirable reaction in the client. The author also assumes no co-responsibility if work with a client is carried out with reference to the statements in this book.

The Author:
Ingo Michael Simon studied psychology and education and is a hypnotherapist with practices in southwestern Germany and Switzerland. With the help of hypnosis-supported psychotherapy, he primarily treats people with persistent psychological conditions. His practice focuses on anxiety disorders, pathological compulsions, and psychosomatic illnesses. His therapeutic offerings mainly include classical and modern hypnosis applications and the dreamland therapy he developed himself.

Copying, publishing, and sharing with third parties are only permitted with the written consent of the author. Please observe the notes on copyright and usage.

Distribution, publication, and copying in any form are prohibited and subject to damages.

Notes on Copyright and Usage

Copying, publishing, and sharing with third parties is prohibited and only permitted with the written consent of the author. Please observe the following copyright and usage guidelines.

This work has been carefully crafted and created to the best of the author's knowledge and personal experience. It comprises text templates and application guidelines for professional hypnosis sessions. The author is a licensed psychotherapist with extensive experience in psychotherapy, coaching, and personal training using hypnotic techniques and methods. Nevertheless, the author and the publisher assume no liability for the accuracy of information, instructions, and advice, nor for any typographical errors. The author and publisher accept no responsibility or liability for the application of these texts and recommendations with clients or patients, nor for any potential consequences or unexpected reactions. It is expressly noted that the application of therapeutic and advisory techniques and formulations lies solely and entirely within the responsibility of the practitioner. This also applies to adherence to the boundaries of legally regulated medical and therapeutic practices. The fact that a book containing action proposals is freely available for sale does not imply that its application with clients or patients is permitted for everyone.

Copying, publishing, and sharing with third parties are only permitted with the written consent of the author. Please observe the notes on copyright and usage.

Distribution, publication, and copying in any form are prohibited and subject to damages.

Copying, publishing, and sharing with third parties are only permitted with the written consent of the author. Please observe the notes on copyright and usage.

Distribution, publication, and copying in any form are prohibited and subject to damages.

Table of Contents

Introduction	9
#1	11
#2	16
#3	21
#4	27
#5	33
#6	41
#7	46
#8	51
#9	55
#10	61
Overview of All Titles in the Series "Ten Hypnoses"	67

Copying, publishing, and sharing with third parties are only permitted with the written consent of the author. Please observe the notes on copyright and usage.

Distribution, publication, and copying in any form are prohibited and subject to damages.

Copying, publishing, and sharing with third parties are only permitted with the written consent of the author. Please observe the notes on copyright and usage.

Introduction

The series "Ten Hypnoses" is very well known in Germany, Austria, and Switzerland as a collection of texts for therapeutic work and is used by numerous psychotherapeutic practices, doctors, therapists, coaches, and other helping professionals. I am pleased to now be able to offer these texts in other countries as well.

Most therapists have their own methods for inducing and deepening trance as well as for exiting trance. Therefore, I have focused on the main part of the hypnosis. The texts in this book can be integrated as the main part into any hypnosis process.

The texts in this collection use various hypnosis techniques. I will not explain these in detail, as I assume that users have the appropriate training. It is also not necessary to understand the exact structure or functioning of the different parts. The texts can simply be read aloud, and they will have their effect.

Decide for yourself which text best suits your client or patient at any given time. You can also combine passages from different texts. It is not about using all ten hypnoses in sequence. It is a selection of possibilities.

I want to emphasize that books cannot replace therapy. Psychotherapy or other therapeutic treatments involve much more. A careful diagnosis is the necessary basis for deciding on the use of methods, including whether hypnosis or one of my texts should be used. Even in this case, preparatory discussions, follow-up discussions during the session, and of course, a therapeutic concept for the sequence of sessions and the content approaches are essential parts of therapy. This cannot and should not be achieved with a collection of texts.

In any case, I wish you much success in your work and I am pleased if my text templates can contribute in a small way.

Ingo Michael Simon

#1

Establishing Contact and Relief

... ... You have experienced something so dramatic that it threw you off course ... ... You have ... [specifically address what happened ... a serious car accident / a train crash with many fatalities / a terrorist attack with casualties, etc. ...] ... ... experienced ... ... It was an immense threat, you feared for your life ... ... Maybe you didn't feel the fear so clearly at first, only much later ... ... Often, in very threatening situations, we somehow keep going and carry on, perhaps in a state of stress and panic, trying to help ourselves in some way ... ... And later, when it's over, we only really realize what happened and how bad and dangerous it actually was ... ... Then often calm returns and we think everything is somewhat back to normal ... ... Maybe that was initially the case for you ... ... And later, often weeks or months afterward, suddenly anxiety and restlessness come, sweating or nightmares ... ... These are so-called post-traumatic reactions ... ... People often don't understand this because at first everything seemed fine, and then much later a huge blow comes and it feels like the world is collapsing ... ... You experienced it that way and initially didn't connect it to the event from back then ... [better to be specific ... the accident / the train crash / the attack, etc.] ... ... maybe you also felt ashamed and thought you should just keep functioning ... ... But nobody can just brush it off and carry on as before ... ... You need time to process it all and even though you have learned to deal with a lot on your own and to endure, you also know that you are allowed to process it calmly and especially with help ... ... that's why you're here ... ... But maybe a part of you still secretly believes that this would be a weakness ... ... Sometimes we even believe that about ourselves without being aware of it ... ...

Self-Forgiveness and Comfort

... ... You would have needed help and comfort immediately, even if you weren't aware of it yourself ... ... Today you help yourself and also seek help to process all this ... ... and now you first find comfort within yourself ... ... This is an important step, so imagine hugging yourself and telling yourself internally that you want to help yourself ... ... just as you would tell another person whom you would help ... ... or as you would help a child who reaches out to you ...

... This self-encounter is important and it is also important to feel how well it already works ... ... It is not at all bad if this idea still feels a bit strange ... ... because more and more you will find it pleasant and good to be close to yourself and to comfort yourself ... ... Comfort for all the terrible things you have experienced ... ... And if you feel guilty or think you could have or should have acted differently, then comfort yourself also for wrestling with yourself ... ... You did not cause the drama and you are not responsible for it ... ... You got caught up in it ... ... and with that, you were and are a victim of the things that happened ... ...

Resolution and Self-Agreement

... ... You have decided to face your memory and even more so your feelings ... ... it is never the memories that burden or harm us ... ... not even the feelings harm us, not even the painful ones ... ... They hurt and occupy us ... ... but they leave no scars ... ... It is always only the judgments of our feelings that can harm us ... ... the judgments that others make and our own judgments ... ... when we think that a feeling of fear or startle is a weakness ... ... or that we are weak because we have problems at all ... ... So now you decide not to make these judgments, but to do something that shows much more strength than judgments or fighting against feelings ... ... Today you decide to let your feelings be there ... ... especially the painful feelings ... ... fear or mortal fear ... ... panic ... ... startle ... ... distrust and suspicion that you have felt since then ... ... and precisely the feelings that occupy you the most ... ... whatever they are ... ... Decide to honor them as your feelings and look at them without judgment ... ... then they will dissolve the fastest ... ... then you will find your peace and your freedom ... ... then these feelings will become memories ... ... Memories do not burden you ... ... They help you ... ... because all, really all memories of life lead to greater experience that you can use constructively for yourself and for your future life ... ... even if you would have liked to spare yourself some experiences ... ... They have happened ... ... But you will be free again ... ...

Success and Reinforcement

... ... Now you can rest and enjoy the trance ... ... this peace and relaxation ... ... You have already achieved a lot because you are on a special path ... ... on a special path to yourself, to your very deep feelings ... ... free from judgments and evaluations ... ... free from demands and pressure to perform ... ... just on your path and that is much more than you might have thought ... ... because with this first step it will be much easier for you to really clear up your experiences and experiences ... ... not for others, but above all for yourself ... ... Now you are important ... ... Now it's your turn and that's good ... ... The experiences and pains will find more and more the place of memory in the coming time ... ... As a memory, all events of life remain within us ... ... But if they are just memories, we can use them as experiences for our future life ... ... That is exactly what you are already doing ... ...

#2

Goal Formulation and Will Strengthening

... ... You can soon leave behind the time of threat and fear ... ... because you have dealt with it and are ready to actively and consciously take new paths ... ... You can soon leave behind the time of threat and fear ... ... because you have processed the past events and now want to be free again ...

... ... You can soon leave behind the time of threat and fear ... ... because you are mentally preparing yourself to look forward now ... ... You can soon leave behind the time of threat and fear ... ... because this trance can help you gather new thoughts and new courage ... ... You are free again ... ... You are safe and free ... ...

Mental Alignment

... ... You know that you are now safe again and can look ahead ... ... and therefore you can feel hope and confidence again ... ...

… … You know that you are now safe again and can look ahead … … and therefore you can be happy again in your everyday life … … You know that you are now safe again and can look ahead … … and therefore you can feel more secure every day … …

… … You know that you are now safe again and can look ahead … … and therefore you look forward to taking new paths, new and self-determined paths … … You are free again … … You are safe and free … …

Somatic Orientation (Body Suggestion)

… … Your body now feels truly healing rest and relaxation … … and therefore you also feel that the wounds of the past are healing more and more … …

… … Your body now feels truly healing rest and relaxation … … and therefore the old fear and insecurity are also fading more and more and you are becoming free … …

… … Your body now feels truly healing rest and relaxation … … and therefore you also find strength within you to start anew … …

… … Your body now feels truly healing rest and relaxation … … and therefore you now start self-determined and sovereign into a new life … … You are free again … … You are safe and free … …

Emotional Orientation (Feeling Suggestion)

… … Even the distrust gradually dissolves and you find trust in life again … … and this life is truly worth living for you … … Even the distrust gradually dissolves and you find trust in life again … … and this life is determined only by you … …

… … Even the distrust gradually dissolves and you find trust in life again … … and this life takes place in freedom and dignity … … Even the distrust gradually dissolves and you find trust in life again … … and this life belongs only to you … … You are free again … … You are safe and free … …

Behavioral Alignment

… … You go your way at your own pace, in your own time … … because this way you free yourself from the past and move forward optimistically … …

… … You go your way at your own pace, in your own time … … because this way you overcome the events of the past and find peace … …You go your way at your own pace, in your own time … … because this way you recognize that your environment is safe again … …

… … You go your way at your own pace, in your own time … … because this way you adjust to new freedom and new opportunities … … You are free again … … You are safe and free … …

Reinforcement

… … You now reclaim your life step by step … … and with it your self-confidence and self-determination … …

… … You now reclaim your life step by step … … and again and again you find your sovereignty and strength and move forward courageously … …

… … You now reclaim your life step by step … … because you are the most important person in your life … …

… … Fear fades away … … The past is over … … You start anew … … You are the most important person in your life … … You are the most important person in your life … …

#3

Preparation

... ... You have experienced something terrible ... [best to be specific ... an accident / an act of violence / a combat mission / a police operation / a shootout ...] ... and this experience has thrown you off course ... ... not immediately, at first you thought you would handle it quite well ... ... you just kept going and functioning ... ... You gathered all your strength, maybe intuitively and without feeling the effort ... ... Maybe you were used to it or it was just your routine to keep going and carry on ... ... But then the uncertainty came slowly ... ... You felt uneasy, were suspicious and somehow afraid ... ... You couldn't explain it to yourself, but you know it has to do with the experiences ... [again, be specific, please ...] ... Usually, it is the case that changes happen weeks after such an incident ... ... But you are here and listening to this hypnosis because you want to overcome this trauma ... ... And an important step in overcoming such drastic experiences is turning towards yourself ... ... and this means a genuine, honest, and above all a deep turning towards yourself ... ... towards your feelings ... ... but also towards self-acceptance and self-love, because only in peace with yourself can you overcome this trauma, but the good thing is ... ... in peace with yourself the trauma then inevitably dissolves ... ... because self-love overcomes all pain ... ... self-love frees from all obstacles ... ... and that is exactly what this hypnosis helps you with ... ... that is exactly what I help you with ... ... in finding and strengthening your self-love, because you are not to blame for the events and consequences that have arisen from them ... ... It was fate or coincidence ... ... But today marks a turning point in your life ... ... And for this change, you say and feel inside yourself ... ...

Self-Acceptance / Self-Acceptance

... ... I am close to myself and feel secure within me ... ...

... ... and security is what I need most right now ... ...

... ... {about 5-10 seconds of silence} ...

... ... I am close to myself and feel secure within me ... ...

... ... and security is what helps me best right now ... ...

… … {about 5-10 seconds of silence} …

… … I am close to myself and feel secure within me … …

… … and security carries me back to a self-confident life …

… … {about 5-10 seconds of silence} …

… … I am close to myself and feel secure within me … …

… … and in this security, I let go of fear and insecurity in peace … …

… … {about 5-10 seconds of silence} …

… … I am close to myself and feel secure within me … …

… … and I feel that I am one with myself and come to terms with myself … …

… … {about 5-10 seconds of silence} …

Self-Forgiveness / Self-Forgiving

… … I accept that I need a break for myself and my feelings

… … because I have realized that this is how I can free myself from the feeling of guilt … …

… … {about 5-10 seconds of silence} …

… … I accept that I need a break for myself and my feelings

… … because I have realized that I am truly innocent … …

… … {about 5-10 seconds of silence} …

… … I accept that I need a break for myself and my feelings … …

… … because I have realized that the past cannot be changed … …

… … {about 5-10 seconds of silence} …

… … I accept that I need a break for myself and my feelings

… … because I have realized that every experience makes me stronger … …

… … {about 5-10 seconds of silence} …

… … I accept that I need a break for myself and my feelings

… … and I feel that I am one with myself and come to terms with myself … … {about 5-10 seconds of silence} …

Self-Love

… … I now take care of myself lovingly and comfort myself … … … … and this self-love makes me strong for all the challenges of life … …

… … {about 5-10 seconds of silence} …

… … I now take care of myself lovingly and comfort myself

… … and this self-love also helps me to overcome crises and lows … …

… … {about 5-10 seconds of silence} …

… … I now take care of myself lovingly and comfort myself

… … and this self-love makes me a satisfied person … …

… … {about 5-10 seconds of silence} …

… … I now take care of myself lovingly and comfort myself

… … and this self-love is a valuable part of me … …

… … {about 5-10 seconds of silence} …

… … I now take care of myself lovingly and comfort myself

… … and I feel that I am one with myself and come to terms with myself … … {about 5-10 seconds of silence} …

#4

Introduction of the Special

… … You have had a burdensome time … … You have freed yourself and want to live in peace and quiet again … … You want to be strong and confident again to shape your life with confidence and without fear … … free from fear … … free from distrust … … free from startle and restlessness … … just calm and relaxed … … Of course, it is not so easy and memories naturally remain … … But … … you have detached yourself from the past … … Maybe we could already say … … You have freed yourself in your feelings and you have made a decision … … or it is not quite done yet and … … You go forward confidently … … with the goal of achieving even more … … You decide that you want to live free and calm again … … to experience and shape a completely normal everyday life again … … You surely know what hypnosis can do … … Maybe you think … … This hypnosis is an important step in liberation … … because you are convinced or consider it possible that … … this hypnosis helps to experience inner and outer peace again … … or you wait a little longer ... ... You decide best ... ... yourself, how the effect of hypnosis is, because ... ... You experience it every day ... ... as soon as you are awake again ... ... Maybe you can soon confirm ... ... These suggestions help you in the liberation and renewal of your life ... ... or you come to a different result ... ... who knows, but we will see and experience it ... ... You will experience it ... ...

Letting Go of the Disturbing/Neutralization

... ... During this terrible event ... [better specify: During your accident / During the attack / During your mission, etc. ...] ... you had terrible fear/death fear ... ... Imagine ... ... You are completely free from fear ... ... Maybe it is actually a long time ago or you can't quite embrace the thought now, but at least you can imagine it ... ... and if it were so, you could say ... ... You are self-confident and strong and you trust ... ... because you are no longer afraid and are strong ... ...

... ... In this state and feeling, you could also easily claim ... ... You feel hope and confidence again ... ... because it would be completely clear to you ... ... You have overcome the terrible experiences [better specify: the accident / the tsunami, etc. ...] and ... ... You are ready for a contented life again ... ... That would be possible ... ...

... ... And maybe it is already possible or partly possible and soon you will realize ... ... Yes, you are really free from fear ... ... Then many things become easier because freed from the old fear, you stand at a point where you can say ... ... Now you trust people and life again ... ... But you have time ... ... You are freer, and you have already overcome the captivity of restlessness and fear ... ... Danger is past ... ... A new life begins and ... ... you decide for yourself ... ... what you want to do with your new life ... ...

Building the New

... ... You have certainly heard something like ... ... Deep inside you lies a very special strength ... ... or ... ... Deep inside, there is no fear and no insecurity ... ... Maybe it's true, if we look very, very deep into your emotions, behind the fear, and ... ... deep inside, there is courage and confidence, peace and trust and ... ...

... ... Maybe there was also a time before when you lived strongly and self-determinedly or decided ... ... Possibly there was a time when it was clear ... ... You definitely determine your life ... ... because it was also clear ... ... You are strong enough to defend yourself ... and ... You are so self-confident that you overcome difficult times well ... ... Back then, maybe it was certain ... ... You are the most important and the strongest person in your life ... ... and today you remember it ... ... or it is about taking and feeling this standpoint now ... ...

... ... Everything has a beginning and it is never too late to start anew ... ... if it goes easily, then you think ... ... That goes really quickly ... ... if it is more difficult, you rather think ... ... It should go faster ... ... because you long for a free and peaceful life ... ...

... ... But here and today you don't need to achieve anything ... ... In trance, many things happen unnoticed and quietly and suddenly we see ... ... Everything is solved by itself ... ... We are amazed and realize ... ... It really works ... ...

Stabilization and Success of the New

... ... You have also heard clear suggestions in the words you heard, but maybe you just let them be and didn't realize how they work ... ... you might have thought ... ... The suggestions you heard should work optimally ... ... and how they work ... ... doesn't matter to you, because the main thing is ... ... They work and free you ... ...

... ... You are right ... ... because in trance you don't have to do anything ... ... You just have to allow them ... ... and that's easy ... ... You relaxed and found your way into the trance ... ... maybe enjoying the peace and relaxation of your body ... ... That's what matters ... ... You don't have to do more ... ... just rest ... ...

... ... As soon as you can recognize the effect of the suggestions in your awake everyday life, you know ... ... Now you are really free ... ... and ... ... Now a free and peaceful life begins, a completely normal and natural life ... ... because then the effect has already fully unfolded and ... ... your goal is achieved ... ... That could be tomorrow or the day after tomorrow ... ... or a little clearer every coming day of your life ... ...

... ... And when you have experienced this success yourself, you will surely also encourage others who are on such a path and tell them ... ... You too experience liberation and freedom ... ... because ... ... Clear suggestions simply work best ... ... Maybe you also tell these people ... ... You will be free and can enjoy your life again ... ... because you know that your decision for the trance was the right path and also want to invite others to go their right path ... ... so that they can say for themselves ... ... Every person can influence and optimize their life themselves ... ... just like you ... ... just like you ... ...

#5

Introduction of the Special

... ... You are here because you want to position yourself strongly and confidently in your new life ... ... That is your goal ... ... You want to be free and without fear ... ... You want to take your life into your own hands and shape it self-determined ... ... So accept the following suggestions, and you will recognize for yourself which you can agree with the most ... ... Clear suggestions that somehow sound familiar and therefore very good usually work the strongest ... [hidden reminder of the previous session with hidden instructions] ... These are the really best suggestions ... ... [hidden instruction to the following suggestions] ...

... You have ... detached yourself from the past ... [5-10 seconds pause] ...

... You have freed yourself in your feelings ... [5-10 seconds pause] ...

... You have made a ... decision ... [5-10 seconds pause] ...

... You go forward ... confidently ... [5-10 seconds pause] ...

... You decide yourself that you want to live ... free and calm again ... [5-10 seconds pause] ...

... This hypnosis ... is an important step of liberation ... [5-10 seconds pause] ...

... This hypnosis helps you ... to experience inner and outer peace again ... [5-10 seconds pause] ...

... You experience it ... every day ... [5-10 seconds pause] ...

... These suggestions help you in the ... renewal of your life ... [5-10 seconds pause] ...

... You have ... detached yourself from the past ... [5-10 seconds pause] ...

... You have freed yourself in your feelings ... [5-10 seconds pause] ...

... You have made a ... decision ... [5-10 seconds pause] ...

... You go forward ... confidently ... [5-10 seconds pause] ...

... You decide yourself that you want to live ... free and calm again ... [5-10 seconds pause] ...

... This hypnosis ... is an important step of liberation ... [5-10 seconds pause] ...

... This hypnosis helps you ... to experience inner and outer peace again ... [5-10 seconds pause] ...

... You experience it ... every day ... [5-10 seconds pause] ...

... These suggestions help you in the ... renewal of your life ... [5-10 seconds pause] ...

Letting Go of the Disturbing/Neutralization

... You are completely ... free from fear ... [5-10 seconds pause] ...

... You are self-confident and strong and ... you trust ... [5-10 seconds pause] ...

... You feel ... hope and confidence again ... [5-10 seconds pause] ...

... You have overcome the terrible experiences ... [5-10 seconds pause] ...

... You have ... [the accident/the tsunami, etc.] ... overcome ... [5-10 seconds pause] ...

... You are ready ... for a contented life again ... [5-10 seconds pause] ...

... Yes, you are really ... free from fear ... [5-10 seconds pause] ...

... Now you trust ... people and life again ... [Now please about 30 seconds pause] ...

... You are completely ... free from fear ... [5-10 seconds pause] ...

... You are self-confident and strong and ... you trust ... [5-10 seconds pause] ...

... You feel ... hope and confidence again ... [5-10 seconds pause] ...

... You have overcome the terrible experiences ... [5-10 seconds pause] ...

... You have ... [the accident/the tsunami, etc.] ... overcome ... [5-10 seconds pause] ...

... You are ready ... for a contented life again ... [5-10 seconds pause] ...

... Yes, you are really ... free from fear ... [5-10 seconds pause] ...

... Now you trust ... people and life again ... [Now please about 30 seconds pause] ...

Building the New

... Deep inside you ... lies a very special strength ... [5-10 seconds pause] ...

... Deep inside ... there is no fear and no insecurity ... [5-10 seconds pause] ...

... There is only courage and confidence ... peace and trust ... [5-10 seconds pause] ...

... You are strong ... enough to assert yourself ... [5-10 seconds pause] ...

... You are so self-confident ... that you overcome difficult times well ... [5-10 seconds pause] ...

... You are the most important and the strongest person ... in your life ... [5-10 seconds pause] ...

... Today you remember ... your strength ... [5-10 seconds pause] ...

... It ... works really ... quickly ... [5-10 seconds pause] ...

... And suddenly everything is ... solved by itself ... [5-10 seconds pause] ...

... It really works ... ... Now ... [Now please about 30 seconds pause] ...

... Deep inside you ... lies a very special strength ... [5-10 seconds pause] ...

... Deep inside ... there is no fear and no insecurity ... [5-10 seconds pause] ...

... There is only courage and confidence ... peace and trust ... [5-10 seconds pause] ...

... You are strong ... enough to assert yourself ... [5-10 seconds pause] ...

... You are so self-confident ... that you overcome difficult times well ... [5-10 seconds pause] ...

... You are the most important and the strongest person ... in your life ... [5-10 seconds pause] ...

... Today you remember ... your strength ... [5-10 seconds pause] ...

... It ... works really ... quickly ... [5-10 seconds pause] ...

... And suddenly everything is ... solved by itself ... [5-10 seconds pause] ...

... It really works ... ... Now ... [Now please about 30 seconds pause] ...

Stabilization and Success of the New

... The suggestions you heard ... work optimally ... [5-10 seconds pause] ...

... You just have to ... allow them ... that's what matters ... [5-10 seconds pause] ...

... Now ... you are really free ... Now ... only you decide ... [5-10 seconds pause] ...

... Your goal is ... achieved ... [5-10 seconds pause] ...

... You also experience liberation and ... freedom ... [5-10 seconds pause] ...

... You live free and in peace ... Now ... [Now please about 30 seconds pause] ...

... The suggestions you heard ... work optimally ... [5-10 seconds pause] ...

... You just have to ... allow them ... that's what matters ... [5-10 seconds pause] ...

... Now ... you are really free ... Now ... only you decide ... [5-10 seconds pause] ...

... Your goal is ... achieved ... [5-10 seconds pause] ...

... You also experience liberation and ... freedom ... [5-10 seconds pause] ...

... You live free and in peace ... Now ... [Now please about 30 seconds pause] ...

#6

Goal Formulation and Will Strengthening

... ... Today you find deep rest in this trance and deep within yourself ... ... because that is the quickest way to find inner freedom, which also frees you externally ... ...

... ... You are determined to listen to and let all suggestions take effect ... ... because that is the quickest way to find inner freedom, which also frees you externally ... ...

... ... You are ready to take in helpful words into your deep inner self ... ... because that is the quickest way to find inner freedom, which also frees you externally ... ...

... ... Today you open yourself to a new path of helpful hypnosis ... ... because that is the quickest way to find inner freedom, which also frees you externally ... ...

Mental Alignment

... ... You know that freedom begins with a free thought in your head ... ... and with this thought, you succeed again and again in shedding inner burdens and moving forward freely ... ...

... ... You know that you are safe again and that everything is alright ... ... and with this thought, you succeed again and again in shedding inner burdens and moving forward freely ... ...

... ... You know that only you have the right to determine your life ... ... and with this thought, you succeed again and again in shedding inner burdens and moving forward freely ... ...

... ... You know that your life belongs to you, only to you ... ... and with this thought, you succeed again and again in shedding inner burdens and moving forward freely ... ...

... ... You are the most important person in your life ... ...

Somatic Orientation (Body Suggestion)

... ... The outer posture of the body reflects the inner attitude ... ... and therefore you succeed in radiating and feeling strength and self-confidence ... ...

... ... Your body can immediately adopt a strong and confident posture and it does ... ... and therefore you succeed in radiating and feeling strength and self-confidence ... ...

... ... Your body is already adopting a really stable and strong posture ... ... and therefore you succeed in radiating and feeling strength and self-confidence ... ...

... ... Your body adopts this stable posture in your everyday life, every day ... ... and therefore you succeed in radiating and feeling strength and self-confidence ... ...

... ... You are the most important person in your life ... ...

Emotional Orientation

... ... You trust your instinct, which warns you of real dangers ... ... and therefore you protect yourself from further dangers by seeking and allowing help ... ...

… … You owe nothing to anyone else, only to yourself … … and therefore you protect yourself from further dangers by seeking and allowing help … …

… … You deserve to live free from fear … … and therefore you protect yourself from further dangers by seeking and allowing help … …

… … Deep inside you find courage and trust … … and therefore you protect yourself from further dangers by seeking and allowing help … …

… … You are the most important person in your life … …

Behavioral Alignment

… … You overcome your fear and find strength and courage within you … … You say yes to your free life and peacefully close the past … [better: end the inner tsunami, etc.] …

… … You are determined to decide for yourself about your future … … You say yes to your free life and peacefully close the past … [better: end the inner tsunami, etc.] …

… … You walk forward with trust and courage … … You say yes to your free life and peacefully close the past … [better: end the inner tsunami, etc.] …

… … You know that it is time to be free again … … You say yes to your free life and peacefully close the past … [better: end the inner tsunami, etc.] …

… … You are the most important person in your life … …

Reinforcement

… … The words you heard work deeper and deeper … … and therefore you overcome the fear and distrust and continue on your own path … … You recognize more clearly every day that you did not bear any guilt during the disaster … [better … during the accident/ during the police operation/ during the attack, etc.] … but were a victim yourself … … and therefore you overcome fear and distrust and continue on your own path … …

… … As soon as you are fully awake again, you recognize even more that you finally want to be free … … and therefore you overcome the fear and distrust and continue on your own path … … You decide about your life alone … … You free yourself from everything that hurts and oppresses you ... ... You free yourself and you stay free ... ... You are and stay free ... ...

#7

Preparation

... ... Today you want to overcome and let go of old feelings of guilt ... ... Feelings of guilt that were never your own, true feelings ... ... You yourself were and are the victim ... ... You have experienced something terrible ... ... You have ... [name specific event: ... a serious accident / an act of violence / an attack / an earthquake, etc.] ... experienced and you couldn't prevent it ... ... You were surprised by this event and above all ... ... It was not your fault ... ... In acts of violence or attacks, the perpetrators are always responsible, and only them ... ... in natural disasters and accidents, sometimes no one is directly responsible ... ... It's often a chain of many circumstances and events ... ... You are innocent anyway ... ... But a part of you believes that you could have acted differently to protect yourself or others ... ... You accuse yourself, but it is time for you to acquit yourself ... ... You have sought and found help, you have allowed help ... ... So you find help again today ... ... with an instance you can believe in or invest hope and trust in ... ...

Maybe you want to find help with a guardian angel or with Jesus ... ... with an inner friend or with your subconscious ... ... or with yourself ... ... Whoever listens to you, your inner self also listens to you ... ... So maybe you say ... ...

Neutralization

... ... Dear Self in the Mirror / Dear God / Dear Guardian Angel / Dear Subconscious ... ... I know that I am innocent because I have recognized and understood that perpetrators are always responsible for their actions ... ... But I am not a perpetrator, I am a victim ... ... Maybe I was in the wrong place at the wrong time ... ... However it came about that I got caught up or drawn into this accident/attack/etc ... ... I didn't choose it ... ... But it happened as it did ... ... and again and again I thought I could have done something differently ... ... Maybe I could have stopped it ... ... No matter how impossible that sounds, a part of me feels partly responsible for what happened ... ... My mind knows that this is not true, but I want to internalize it deeper in my feelings ... ... Please help me to feel truly innocent and free deep in my feelings ... ... With your help, I can and will do it, I know that ... ... Dear Self in the Mirror / Dear God / Dear Guardian Angel / Dear Subconscious ... ... Help me let go of the old guilt that was never my own ... ... Mind and feeling should go hand in hand ... ... innocent and free ... ...

Reorientation

... ... Dear Self in the Mirror / Dear God / Dear Guardian Angel / Dear Subconscious ... ... I know that I am the one who must take my life into my own hands because I am responsible for the constructive design of my life ... ... I can and want to gladly bear this responsibility, and with your support, I can do it even faster ... ... I am ready to open myself to the opportunities and possibilities of life again and look forward ... ... I know that I can process the past and understand more and more what actually happened to me ... ... Dear Self in the Mirror / Dear God / Dear Guardian Angel / Dear Subconscious ... ... Please show me how to process the past and look forward confidently at the same time ... ...

Attention, Perception, and Self-Acceptance

... ... Dear Self in the Mirror / Dear God / Dear Guardian Angel / Dear Subconscious ... ... I know that I must accept myself as I am ... ... how I feel and think ... ... I want to accept myself, with all my strengths and with all my weaknesses, because I recognize more and more that both sides are special ... ... What I considered guilty weaknesses are in truth just traits and characteristics of mine ... ... On the one hand, I want to become free and not feel guilty anymore, because I am not guilty ... ... On the other hand, and this is important, I want to acknowledge that these feelings of guilt have accompanied me and thus were also a part of me and certainly, I could also learn a lot in this time ... ... Above all, I have learned that I do not have to bear the guilt of others ... ... and that sometimes no one bears any guilt ... ... I have understood that I cannot alleviate terrible events with my own feelings of guilt ... ... So I want to try to live with all my traits and make the best of myself and my possibilities ... ... in a life without feelings of guilt ... ... in a free life ... ... I know I can do that with your support ... ...

Outlook and Self-Care

... ... Dear Self in the Mirror / Dear God / Dear Guardian Angel / Dear Subconscious ... ... Please help me to treat myself considerately ... ... especially when I do accuse myself or when I feel that I occasionally still have feelings of guilt, although my mind knows that I am innocent ... ... Then I want to be patient with myself and trust that I can let go of these feelings of guilt very soon ... ... For your support, I thank you and also myself because I know that a part of your help is always my self-help ... ... Help from my deep inner self for me ... ...

Reinforcement

... ... So ... ... Now you can rest a bit because you have taken another very important step ... ... You have asked your Self / God / your Guardian Angel / your Subconscious for help and thus also an inner instance within you ... ... So you can trust in double help ... ... So your deepest inner self adjusts to do everything that helps you overcome and let go of old feelings of guilt ... ... So you experience new liberation with every new day ... ... So you can shape your new life every new day and be free ... ... really free ... ... You are and stay free ... ...

#8

Preparation

... ... Today you want to overcome the anxiety, uncertainty, and mistrust of the recent time and turn back to life ... ... a free and self-determined life that you can enjoy ... ... and live in naturalness and freedom ... ... You want to actively and consciously face everyday life again and accept it with all its challenges ... ... with everything that makes up your life and plays a role in it ... ... So you find the way to your deep feelings and thus the way to your potential and new trust ... ... Trust in yourself ... ... in your feelings, in your instincts ... ... Your subconscious helps you with this because it hears and understands every word I say ... ... And every word you can agree with becomes your own word ... ... Then it is as if you are saying all these words yourself or saying them inwardly ... ... So you are the one who says ... ...

Self-Encounter and Self-Care

… … I turn my gaze inward, feel into the depths to feel my true feelings and find trust in life and my surroundings again … … and my inner self opens trustingly and lets me recognize my feelings better … …

… … I want to find hope and trust again in the depths of my feelings and at the same time feel safe … … and gently and trustingly my inner self meets me and invites me to look deeper and deeper … …

… … With curiosity and satisfaction, I find myself in my inner center and experience there confidence, self-confidence, and hope … … and my inner center, this place of my feelings, comes to me with warmth and peace … …

Self-Acceptance and External Impact

… … I am ready to overcome the time of anxiety and isolation and listen to the trustful in me and open myself to the people around me … … and also my fellow human beings meet me trustingly and friendly on my way … …

… … I accept that I myself slowly and carefully find my way back to normality, to my need for social contacts and exchange with other people ... ... and I am sure that I encounter understanding and support in my environment ...

... ... I trust my instincts and my feelings and I know they warn me early of foreseeable dangers and threats ... ... and I rejoice in the freedom and honesty I can recognize and experience in my surroundings ... ...

Behavioral Orientation and External Impact

... ... I meet my fellow human beings friendly and open and at the same time allow myself to set boundaries and maintain constructive distance ... ... and I also accept the boundaries of other people who accept mine ... ...

... ... I open myself confidently again to encounters with others in my everyday life and look forward to new acquaintances ... ... and every day, I also meet benevolent and friendly people in my everyday life ... ...

... ... I am open and at the same time allow myself to draw clear boundaries and preserve my freedom ... ... and my fellow human beings recognize and respect these boundaries and accept my self-determination ... ...

Success and Reinforcement

... ... I am sure that by looking inward, I find myself again above all, and that it helps me to stand by myself more and more and trust myself ... ... and I experience acceptance and trust daily in the reactions of my fellow human beings ... ...

... ... I trust that I am strong enough to face everyday life and all its challenges ... ... and I experience respect and appreciation from my environment and from people who understand and accompany my path ... ...

... ... In my uniqueness and in my personal development, I am an asset to my environment because I take responsibility for my life again, which I constructively and consciously shape ... ... and my fellow human beings are an asset to my own life because I can learn from them and also appreciate and accept their uniqueness ... ...

#9

Ideomotorics refers to the phenomenon that our body follows our feelings and thoughts with movements. In everyday life, this following is shown as body posture, muscle tension, and movement patterns of a person, which naturally change with the mood and thoughts. In trance, ideomotor signals can be used to obtain information that the client cannot actively communicate. For example, the subconscious can answer questions with an agreed finger signal. Naturally, ideomotor responses can also be used suggestively, for example, in arm levitation and catalepsy. Such an approach, which I also use in the following text, strengthens trust in hypnosis and one's own ability to change and thus promotes therapy.

Goal Formulation and Preparation

... ... Today you want to let go of the tormenting memory ... ... You want to free yourself from the images and impressions that have accompanied you for so long ... ...

You have tried that many times, but then the images came back because you couldn't really imagine that the feelings attached to them would finally dissolve ... ... because you couldn't really believe that they would actually get smaller and disappear ... ... Today you can get special help, help from your subconscious ... ... maybe you wonder how that can work exactly ... ... how that can work exactly ... ... so this hypnosis becomes an exciting journey for you ... ... We can ask your subconscious if it can do that ... ... we can ask it to show you that it can let go of the burdensome images and feelings ... ... because it actually can ... ... So let's go ... ...

Establishing Catalepsy

... ... Now focus on your goal of letting go of the fear-laden and burdensome images ... ... Imagine how nice it would be if that were already done ... ... how good it feels when just memories are there that you can easily bear ... ... Place your hands loosely beside your body ... ... with the palms up ... ... Let your hands be completely loose and above all ... ... Do not help me with it, because you don't need to shake off or drive away anything ... ... Your subconscious lets go ... ... Your subconscious lets go of disturbing and burdensome images and exchanges them for memories that you can easily bear ... ... maybe even for the same images, just completely without fear and without terror ... ... Now do nothing ... ... Take in my words and do not help me with it ... ... Your subconscious can and will act for you ... ... Your deep inner self can and will let go of the painful images and feelings for you ... ... Formulate this wish, your goal, in your mind and tell your subconscious ... ... Now let go of the painful memories and replace them with harmless memories ... ... All images and feelings are stored in your body and flow into your open hands ... ... all fear feelings dissolve and now flow into your open hands, which may feel heavier because of it ... ... That is completely fine because you will let go of the fear very soon ... ... All guilt feelings flow into your hands ... ... right and left ... ... and make the hands heavier ... ... Every distrust flows into the hands ... ... right and left ... ... and makes the hands heavier ... ... good so ... ... You are doing exactly right ... ... Your hands are getting heavier and more immobile ... ... heavy as lead and completely immobile because they now hold these old feelings that arose during the dramatic event ... the accident / the tsunami / the hurricane / the shootout ... ...

Only your hands hold these feelings and the images associated with them ... ... the hands are getting heavier and heavier ... ... because they hold these heavy feelings ... ... and everything is fine because now the change can begin ... ...

Ideomotor Task

... ... Now your subconscious lets go of these painful feelings and thereby also the connection between the feelings and the images of the memory ... ... Your subconscious can do that ... ... and thereby your hands become lighter and they start to turn ... ... your hands now become lighter and lighter because the painful feelings detach from the images of the memory and because you let go of these feelings ... ... You recognize this because your hands turn as you empty the full hands ... ... The more your subconscious lets go, the more your hands turn, which become lighter and lighter ... ... Your hands become lighter and turn ... ... They become lighter and turn ... ... [Wait for the complete turn of both hands!] ...

[Please try to be patient if it takes a while for the hands to turn. Ideomotor signals are reliable signs, similar to kinesiology muscle tests. Here we work with a mixture of suggestive request and ideomotor communication. When you repeatedly say ... Your hands turn ... it has a suggestive effect and the ideomotor response follows. By assuming that this is connected with letting go of the painful feelings and the connection to the images of the traumatic event, a coupling occurs in the unconscious. The subconscious confirms this by turning the hands. If letting go were not possible, it would not be logical to turn the hands. If the turn happens only because of the suggestion, it is still proof of letting go for the mind because it was "agreed upon" this way. If the mind is convinced, the goal is almost achieved. Please try it out. The effect may surprise you.]

Resolving Catalepsy

... ... Your subconscious has detached the painful feelings of fear and insecurity and distrust from the images of the memory and let go and made your hands light again ... ... you have achieved a lot and will feel this new freedom in your everyday life ... ... Your hands are now light and movable again because they are open to new things ... ... The memory of the accident / the tsunami / the shootout ... ... remains as images that you can look at with distance and can easily bear ... ... But you have let go of the painful and fearful feelings today ... ... and deep inside your subconscious lets go of these feelings again and again ... ... so they do not come up again ... ... You do not need them anymore, your subconscious confirmed that because that is why it let go of them and only for that reason ... ... because you absolutely do not need them anymore and can really be free ... ... Your subconscious gives you back full control of your hands, which can feel good ... ... You can check it ... ... Simply move your hands and fingers ... ...

Reinforcement (Posthypnotic Task)

... ... Your subconscious was able to free you from old feelings today ... ... by turning your hands ... ... and you can do it too ... ... You can easily repeat it in your awake everyday life ... ... If you ever have the thought that the images of your memory come along with painful or oppressive feelings that you do not want to have ... ... then you simply turn your hands consciously ... ... You simply turn both hands once and remember the letting go ... ... and thereby your deep inner self immediately remembers the letting go and lets go again with and for you ... ... just like today ... ... just as easily and quickly as today ... ...

#10

Arriving in the Land of Dreams

... ... There is a magical place deep in your imagination ... ... a place only you can reach ... ... It is a place where memories dwell and wait for you to look at them and learn from your own experience ... ... This place is the land of dreams ... ... The dreams there are like dreams at night ... ... with unexpected images and impressions that are suddenly there ... ... because feelings are suddenly there and find a way to you ... ... Maybe you know that dreams at night are pictorial feelings ... ... So it is also in the land of dreams ... ... So it is in every daydream and in every fantasy ... ... Imagine being there ... ... deep in your feelings ... ... deep in your imagination ... ... deep in the land of dreams ... ... and wait curiously and openly for the images of the dream that shows your feelings and memories ...

Confrontation, Clarification, and Creative Reorientation

... ... You stand outside, in nature ... ... at the edge of a deep valley ... ... You stand on a path that leads into the deep valley ... ... It is the valley of silence ... ... Down in the valley, it is quiet, and only the moment counts ... ... You start walking, and your goal is to reach this place of silence ... ... But there are so many feelings in you that your thoughts circle, and you constantly think ... ... about guilt and responsibility ... ... about fear and disaster ... ... and about how you can find peace and experience a completely normal everyday life the quickest ... ... You have experienced something terrible ... [specify ... an earthquake / a serious accident / a combat mission / a terrorist attack, etc.] ... and since then, you can hardly find peace ... ... But that is possible today ... ... Finding peace ... ... peace and freedom ... ... For that, you go into the deep valley ... ... Your path leads down over three levels ... ... and on each level, you make peace with a feeling in you ... ... Making peace means accepting the feeling and letting it out ... ... and then becoming free again ... ...

... ... On the first level, you encounter fear ... ... It appears as a gray figure wrapped in a cloak and covering its face ... ... That's how it was during the earthquake / accident / combat mission / terrorist attack ... ... Suddenly it happened, and everything went very quickly ... ... Everything was different than you thought, and you couldn't do much yourself ... ... Now you are safe, and now the fear stands as a gray figure before you ... ... shy and cautious itself ... ... and you dive into your memory, but only as far as you can bear it well because the most important thing now is the encounter here, in the land of dreams ... ... Here you do something that you might not have planned or expected this way ... ... You reach out to the fear ... ... It is your fear that stands here ... ... It is your fear that wanders around aimlessly and without a goal in the land of dreams, in the land of your own feelings ... ... homeless and without a goal ... ... So you reach out to the fear ... ... and with that, you accept this feeling as your feeling ... ... This feeling of fear that could burden you so much in its aimless search and its lostness now gets a home in you ... ... All feelings that are in us and belong to us need a home ... ... And suddenly, this gray figure dissolves into light blue light before your eyes ... ... It begins to glow light blue and finally dissolves ... ... and finds a home in you as a memory ... ... only as a memory and as an experience ... ... and you feel freer ... ...

... ... On the second level, you meet distrust ... ... Distrust also stands as a gray figure before you ... ... aimless and homeless ... ... and you remember that you have been very suspicious and wary recently ... ... You often expected disaster, thought something would happen again or that fate would catch up with you ... ... You were insecure, and that is quite natural because after all, the events during the earthquake / accident / combat mission / terrorist attack were indeed dramatic and formative ... ... But this homeless feeling wanders around in the depths of your emotions and drives you around ... ... it created this unrest that you have felt so often and for so long ... ... like the fear, it has contributed to your insecurity and your despondency ... ... But just as you dissolved the fear, you can also dissolve the distrust ... ... So you can also reach out to this feeling ... ... You can do it because it's not about reaching out to an event or a perpetrator or responsible person, but to your own feeling ... ... This way, you end the fight against the feeling, and this way, you reconcile with yourself ... ... This feeling of distrust that could burden you so much in its aimless search and its lostness now gets a home in you ... ... All feelings that are in us and belong to us need a home ... ... And suddenly, this gray figure dissolves into light blue light before your eyes ... ... It begins to glow light blue and finally dissolves ... ... and finds a home in you as a memory ... ... only as a memory and as an experience ... ... and you feel freer ... ...

... ... Finally, you come to the third level of depth, and it is already quieter around you ... ... and quieter within you ... ... and there you meet self-love ... ... It meets you as a twin brother/twin sister in red clothes ... ... surrounded by a red aura, a beautiful red glow ... ... You remember that you could hardly feel self-love recently and especially since the earthquake / accident / combat mission / terrorist attack ... ... Fear and insecurity were too great ... ... The images of the memory of this terrible event had occupied you too much ... ... And maybe you also rarely or just not so consciously and actively perceived your self-love before ... ... Today, however ... ... Today you feel it ... ... So you also reach out to self-love, and that feels warm ... ... And you go deeper and deeper into the valley of silence ... ... Self-love accompanies you as your twin brother / your twin sister on this path ... ... You do not walk this path into the depth alone ... ... You do not walk any path alone because your self-love always accompanies you ... ... here, in the land of dreams and also in your everyday life ... ... And together with self-love, you reach the deep valley of silence and enjoy the inner peace ... ...

Mindfulness and Self-Loyalty

... ... At your own pace, in your own time, you walk through the valley of silence and feel deep peace within you ... ... and true self-love ... ... Now everything is alright ... ... In the land of dreams, you are safe and confident ... ... but not only here, also in your awake everyday life, you are confident again and feel this peace and this self-love because the land of dreams is not somewhere ... ... The land of dreams lies deep within you ... ... It has always been there ... ... I am just telling you about it ... ...

Distribution, publication, and copying in any form are prohibited and subject to damages.

Overview of All Titles in the Series "Ten Hypnoses"

Volume 1: Smoking Cessation
Volume 2: Anxiety and Restlessness
Volume 3: Burnout
Volume 4: Reducing Overweight
Volume 5: Coping with the Past
Volume 6: Suicidal Thoughts and Attempts
Volume 7: Psycho-Oncology
Volume 8: Obsessions and Tics
Volume 9: Self-Confidence and Decision-Making
Volume 10: Grief Work
Volume 11: Psychosomatics
Volume 12: Chronic Pain
Volume 13: Depressive Thoughts
Volume 14: Panic Attacks
Volume 15: Domestic Violence, Victim Support
Volume 16: Post-Traumatic Stress
Volume 17: Exam Anxiety and Stage Fright
Volume 18: Anti-Violence Training, Offender Support
Volume 19: Addiction Tendencies
Volume 20: Social Phobia and Fear of Contact
Volume 21: Nail Biting
Volume 22: Self-Awareness and Self-Love
Volume 23: Teeth Grinding and Night Clenching
Volume 24: Feelings of Guilt
Volume 25: Fear in Crowds
Volume 26: Fear of Flying, Aviophobia
Volume 27: Fear in Enclosed Spaces, Claustrophobia
Volume 28: Tinnitus, Ear Noises
Volume 29: Fear of Heights
Volume 30: Neurodermatitis

Copying, publishing, and sharing with third parties are only permitted with the written consent of the author. Please observe the notes on copyright and usage.

Volume 31: Finding Inner Balance
Volume 32: Overcoming Loneliness
Volume 33: Fear of Illness, Hypochondria
Volume 34: Anticipatory Anxiety, Fear of Fear
Volume 35: Jealousy in Relationships
Volume 36: Driving Anxiety
Volume 37: New Start after Separation
Volume 38: Fear of Injections
Volume 39: Heart Anxiety Neurosis
Volume 40: Overcoming Resentment and Anger
Volume 41: Resolving Blockages and Positive Thinking
Volume 42: Stress Reduction, Stress Management
Volume 43: Body Relaxation
Volume 44: Deep Relaxation
Volume 45: Fear of the Dark
Volume 46: Falling Asleep and Staying Asleep
Volume 47: Compulsive Buying
Volume 48: Restless Legs Syndrome
Volume 49: Bulimia
Volume 50: Anorexia
Volume 51: Overcoming Nightmares
Volume 52: Imagined Deformity
Volume 53: Overcoming Distrust, Finding Trust
Volume 54: Processing Failures
Volume 55: Humiliation, Emotional Hurt
Volume 56: Distressing Compassion, Vicarious Suffering
Volume 57: Self-Forgiveness
Volume 58: Self-Awareness, Self-Confidence
Volume 59: Saying No
Volume 60: Assertiveness
Volume 61: Setting Boundaries and Self-Assertion
Volume 62: Decision-Making Ability

Volume 63: Success Orientation
Volume 64: Ruminating, Circular Thinking
Volume 65: Accepting Pregnancy
Volume 66: Birth Preparation
Volume 67: Spiritual Opening
Volume 68: Joy of Life and Inner Lightness
Volume 69: Patience and Inner Peace
Volume 70: Fibromyalgia and Rheumatism
Volume 71: Irritable Bowel Syndrome, Crohn's Disease
Volume 72: Fear of Nausea, Emetophobia
Volume 73: Stuttering and Cluttering, Speech Flow Disorders
Volume 74: Concentration and Knowledge Anchoring
Volume 75: Vitality and Spontaneity
Volume 76: Searching for Meaning and Finding Goals
Volume 77: Life Crises, Life Events
Volume 78: Workaholism, Goal Obsession
Volume 79: Helper Syndrome, Helpless Helpers
Volume 80: Medication Abuse
Volume 81: Gambling Addiction
Volume 82: Internet Addiction, Smartphone Addiction
Volume 83: Hoarding Disorder, Compulsive Collecting
Volume 84: Conspiracy Thoughts, Overvalued Ideas
Volume 85: Fear of Operations and Treatments
Volume 86: Fear of Aging
Volume 87: Travel Anxiety
Volume 88: Anxiety When Urinating, Paruresis
Volume 89: Fear of Intimacy and Togetherness
Volume 90: Fear of Blushing
Volume 91: Coming Out in Homosexuality
Volume 92: Charisma Training
Volume 93: Migraines and Chronic Headaches
Volume 94: Overcoming Allergies, Bronchial Asthma

Volume 95: Normalizing Blood Pressure
Volume 96: Compulsive Perfectionism
Volume 97: Sports Hypnosis, Motivation
Volume 98: Sports Hypnosis, Performance Enhancement
Volume 99: Determination and Focus
Volume 100: Encountering the Inner Child
Volume 101: Cravings, Binge Eating
Volume 102: Stimulating Metabolism
Volume 103: Bipolar Mood Swings
Volume 104: Borderline, Identity Crises
Volume 105: Hypomania, Euphoria, Mania
Volume 106: Restlessness, Agitation
Volume 107: Nervous Breakdown
Volume 108: Adjustment Disorders
Volume 109: Self-Alienation, Depersonalization
Volume 110: Ending Self-Pity
Volume 111: Primary Gain of Illness
Volume 112: Secondary Gain of Illness
Volume 113: Bullying, Victim Support
Volume 114: Letting Go of Envy and Jealousy
Volume 115: Fear of Spiders, Arachnophobia
Volume 116: Fear of Dogs or Cats
Volume 117: Fear of Strangers, Xenophobia
Volume 118: Excessive Worries, Generalized Anxiety
Volume 119: Strengthening Sense of Responsibility
Volume 120: Unrequited Love, Heartache
Volume 121: Work-Life Balance
Volume 122: Letting Go of Unattainable Goals
Volume 123: Allowing and Accepting Help
Volume 124: Letting Go of Adult Children
Volume 125: Tourette Syndrome
Volume 126: Life Changes and New Starts

Volume 127: Accepting Life in a Wheelchair
Volume 128: Understanding and Overcoming Homesickness
Volume 129: Understanding and Overcoming Wanderlust
Volume 130: Dizziness, Meniere's Disease
Volume 131: Overcoming Aggression
Volume 132: Cutting and Self-Harm
Volume 133: Hair Pulling, Trichotillomania
Volume 134: Postpartum Depression
Volume 135: For Relatives of Dementia Patients
Volume 136: Self-Harm, Artificial Disorders
Volume 137: Activating Self-Healing Powers
Volume 138: Preventing Depression Relapse
Volume 139: Reactive Psychoses, Follow-Up
Volume 140: Obsessive Thoughts and Impulses
Volume 141: Compulsive Checking
Volume 142: Compulsive Counting, Symmetry Obsession
Volume 143: Compulsive Washing, Cleanliness Obsession
Volume 144: Compulsive Questioning
Volume 145: Dissociative Paralysis
Volume 146: Phantom Pain
Volume 147: Overcoming Complaining
Volume 148: Hay Fever, Pollen Allergy
Volume 149: Sexual Abuse, Victim Support
Volume 150: Standing Strong Against Sexism, #metoo
Volume 151: Binge Eating
Volume 152: Overcoming Thoughts of Revenge
Volume 153: Detachment from the Aggressor, Stockholm Syndrome
Volume 154: Courage to Separate
Volume 155: Chronic Fatigue, Exhaustion
Volume 156: Fear of the Future, Existential Anxiety
Volume 157: Excessive Worry About Children
Volume 158: Fear of Failure

Volume 159: Ending Distrust and Control
Volume 160: Dejection, Dysphoria
Volume 161: Boreout, Chronic Boredom
Volume 162: Bipolar Disorders, Relapse Prevention
Volume 163: Mania, Relapse Prevention
Volume 164: Nihilism, Feelings of Worthlessness
Volume 165: Thumb Sucking
Volume 166: Being Brave
Volume 167: Being Proud
Volume 168: Overcoming Shyness
Volume 169: Being Able to Delegate Responsibility
Volume 170: Being Able to Show Emotions
Volume 171: Letting Go of Guilt, Victim Support
Volume 172: Processing Guilt, Offender Support
Volume 173: Mood Swings, Cyclothymia
Volume 174: Lack of Drive, Vital Sadness
Volume 175: Hearing Voices with Reality Reference
Volume 176: Confident Communication
Volume 177: Standing Up for Oneself
Volume 178: Taking New Paths
Volume 179: Confident Job Application
Volume 180: No Longer Being Taken Advantage Of
Volume 181: End of Submissiveness
Volume 182: Depressive Numbness
Volume 183: Mood Drops, Affective Incontinence
Volume 184: Mood Instability
Volume 185: Somatoform Disorders
Volume 186: Stomach Ulcer, Psychosomatic
Volume 187: Accepting Amputation
Volume 188: Overcoming and Letting Go of Hatred
Volume 189: Ending Accusations
Volume 190: Allowing Tears, Being Able to Cry

Volume 191: Finding and Sorting Repressed Feelings
Volume 192: Somatoform Pain
Volume 193: Living Autonomously
Volume 194: Anhedonia, Joylessness
Volume 195: Persistent Sadness
Volume 196: Obesity, Food Addiction
Volume 197: Parents of Abused Children
Volume 198: Letting Go and Letting Be
Volume 199: Childhood Sexual Abuse
Volume 200: Fear of Loss

www.ingramcontent.com/pod-product-compliance
Lightning Source LLC
Chambersburg PA
CBHW030454220526
45464CB00006B/2540